Dr. Macklene.C. Jones

EXPECTING WITH COURAGE

'Navigating HIV / AIDS in Pregnancy'

Contents

Introduction

Bringing a child into the world is an amazing and joyful process full of hopes, dreams, and expectations. However, for those living with HIV/AIDS, the path to motherhood can be fraught with new problems and uncertainty. "Expecting with Courage: Navigating Pregnancy with HIV/AIDS," a caring and powerful guide, is intended to help and inspire women on this incredible journey.

Pregnancy should be a time of wonder and celebration, but when HIV/AIDS enters the picture, worry and anxiety may easily overpower the joy. We recognize the concerns and questions that may arise: Is it possible for me to have a healthy pregnancy? Will my child become infected? How will my disease affect my health and the health of my child? Don't worry, you are not alone, dear reader. We hope that the information, skills, and support provided on these pages will help you negotiate the obstacles of HIV/AIDS pregnancy.

We will delve into the various facets of this journey chapter by chapter, providing you with the information you need to make informed decisions and ensure that you receive the best possible treatment. We will discuss the principles of HIV/AIDS and its consequences for pregnancy, including transmission risks and treatment alternatives. We will also explore prenatal care, drugs, nutrition, and emotional well-being to help you manage your health and wellness during this vital time.

Recognizing the significance of developing a support network, we will assist you in navigating the difficult topics around HIV/AIDS disclosure. We will discuss the resources and networks accessible to you for professional help and emotional support, as well as communication with your loved ones. Furthermore, we will enable you to advocate for yourself, ensuring that you are informed of your rights and prepared to plan for life after pregnancy.

We emphasize throughout this book that, while living with HIV/AIDS can bring unique obstacles, it does not define you or limit your ability to enjoy the joys of motherhood. You may embrace this path with courage and hope if you have the correct information, support, and a resilient spirit.

We recognize that each woman's experience is unique, and this book is meant to be a complete reference that speaks to your specific need. Whether you have recently been diagnosed, this book is intended to provide you with knowledge, encouragement, and practical help if you have HIV/AIDS, are planning to conceive, or are already on the path to motherhood.

Above all, we want to reassure you that you have the inner strength to traverse this trip gracefully. As you read "Expecting with Courage: Navigating Pregnancy with HIV/AIDS," may you find comfort, inspiration, and the steadfast belief that parenting is a journey worth embracing, no matter what obstacles you face.

Remember that you are not alone on this journey. Let us go on this changing journey together, full of hope, resilience, and the power of motherly love.

Chapter 1

HIV/AIDS and its Effects on Pregnancy

The Human Immunodeficiency Virus (HIV) discovery and the subsequent rise of acquired immunodeficiency syndrome (AIDS) have had a tremendous impact on individuals, families, and communities all over the world. Significant progress has been made in understanding and managing HIV/AIDS in recent years, converting it from a fatal sickness to a chronic condition that can be effectively treated with the proper treatment and support.

However, the interaction of HIV/AIDS with pregnancy presents particular issues and challenges for women who are pregnant or want to conceive. The goal of this chapter is to provide you with a basic grasp of HIV/AIDS and its consequences for pregnancy. By learning about the consequences of this, you will be better equipped to make informed decisions and take proactive steps to protect your own and your baby's health.

In this chapter, we will look at the following topics in depth:

1.2 A Quick Overview of HIV/AIDS

What is the distinction between HIV and AIDS?

Statistics and Trends on the global impact of HIV/AIDS

Modes of transmission: How does HIV spread?

1.3 HIV/AIDS with Pregnancy: Risks and Factors to Consider

Vertical transmission refers to the possibility of mother-to-child transmission.

Transmission rate influencing factors

Implications for the mother's and Baby's Health

1.4 The Importance of Pregnancy HIV Testing and Diagnosis

The Importance of Early Testing

The following tests are available: Prenatal and postnatal screening

Confidentiality and informed consent are essential.

1.5 Treatment Options and Their Consequences

ART (antiretroviral treatment) during pregnancy: advantages and disadvantages

Side effects and potential dangers

Healthcare Providers' roles in treatment decision-making

Understanding the impact of HIV/AIDS on pregnancy is critical for preserving the mother's and baby's health. You may make informed decisions and engage in proactive healthcare management if you understand the virus, how it spreads, and what treatment options are available.

We advise you to approach the information in the next sections of this chapter with an open mind and a willingness to ask questions. Remember that knowledge is power, and by understanding the complexities of HIV/AIDS and its impacts on pregnancy, you can take charge of your health, encourage a healthy pregnancy, and build the groundwork for a brighter future for both you and your child.

1.2 A Quick Overview of HIV/AIDS

To understand the influence of HIV/AIDS on pregnancy, it is necessary to first understand the virus and its progression to acquired immunodeficiency syndrome (AIDS). This section describes HIV/AIDS, including its description, global impact, and mechanisms of transmission.

HIV, which stands for Human Immunodeficiency Virus, is a virus that affects the immune system, specifically the CD4 cells (also known as Thelper cells), which play an important role in the body's defense against infections. HIV, if left untreated, can gradually weaken the immune system, rendering people more vulnerable to opportunistic infections and some types of malignancies. AIDS, or acquired immunodeficiency syndrome, is the most advanced stage of HIV infection by significant immune system damage and the emergence of particular opportunistic infections or malignancies.

The Global Impact of HIV/AIDS: Since its discovery in the 1980s, HIV/AIDS has become one of the most serious global health issues of our time. As of 2020, the World Health Organization (WHO) predicted that 38 million individuals worldwide were living with HIV/AIDS. The virus's impact varies by geography, with Sub-Saharan Africa being the most severely afflicted. HIV/AIDS, on the other hand, affects people of all ages, genders, and socioeconomic backgrounds.

HIV is primarily spread: By certain body fluids such as blood, sperm, vaginal secretions, and breast milk. The following are the most common modes of transmission:

Sexual intercourse without protection: HIV transmission can occur during anal or oral sex without the use of barrier devices such as condoms.

Sharing infected needles: Sharing needles or other drug paraphernalia with an HIV-positive individual might help the virus spread.

HIV transmission from mother to kid: HIV can be spread from an infected woman to her child during pregnancy, childbirth, or breastfeeding. The probability of mother-to-child transmission, however, can be considerably lowered with adequate measures.

Transmission via blood transfusion or organ transplantation: From an infected donor is still a possibility in some locations, although being rare in resource-rich countries with strong screening standards.

Occupational exposure: Healthcare workers may be exposed to HIV through unintentional needlestick injuries or contact with contaminated blood or body fluids. However, compliance with general measures and post-exposure prophylaxis can minimize this risk.

Understanding the modalities of HIV transmission is critical for implementing preventative measures and adopting safer behaviors to lower the risk of infection or transmission.

Understanding the fundamentals of HIV/AIDS, such as its definition, worldwide effect, and mechanisms of transmission, can better prepare you to understand how it may intersect with pregnancy. This knowledge helps as a basis for making educated decisions and taking proactive measures to protect your and your baby's health. In the parts that follow, we will look at the specific risks and issues connected with HIV/AIDS during pregnancy, as well as the significance of testing and diagnosis.

1.3 HIV/AIDS with Pregnancy: Risks and Factors to Consider

When HIV/AIDS interacts with pregnancy, some additional dangers and considerations must be addressed to preserve the mother's and baby's health and well-being. This section investigates the possible hazards of HIV/AIDS during pregnancy, as well as the factors that can influence transmission rates and health consequences.

Vertical Transmission and the Dangers of Mother-to-Child Transmission

The danger of vertical transmission, which refers to the transmission of the virus from the mother to her child during pregnancy, childbirth, or breastfeeding, is one of the key concerns for HIV-positive moms. Without effective measures, the probability of transmission might range from 15% to 45%. However, with the availability of effective interventions such as antiretroviral therapy (ART) and other antiretroviral therapies (ART), With the right precautions, the risk can be minimized to less than 1%.

Transmission Rate Influencing Factors

Several factors can influence the chance of HIV transmission from mother to child. The maternal viral load (the quantity of HIV in the mother's blood), the presence of other sexually transmitted infections (STIs), the duration of ruptured membranes during labor, the style of birth (vaginal delivery or cesarean section), and breastfeeding practices are among these factors. Understanding these factors and their implications can assist healthcare providers in developing personalized management programs to reduce the risk of transmission.

Implications for Mother and Child Health

HIV/AIDS during pregnancy can have serious consequences for both the mother's and the baby's health. HIV infection may have an impact on the mother's overall health and immunological function, potentially leading to an increased risk of opportunistic infections and problems. Comprehensive prenatal treatment for HIV-positive pregnant women is critical, including regular monitoring of their viral load, CD4 count, and overall health condition.

The biggest concern for the newborn Is the chance of contracting HIV during pregnancy, childbirth, or breastfeeding. Untreated HIV infection in newborns can cause serious health problems and an increased chance of death. However, with the right measures in place, such as maternal ART, obstetric management strategies, and alternate feeding alternatives, the risk of transmission can be considerably decreased, giving the baby a better chance of being HIV-free at birth.

Navigating these dangers and considerations necessitates a team effort from healthcare providers, HIV experts, obstetricians, and the woman herself. Using good medical care, the goal is to give the best possible outcomes for both the mother and the infant by adhering to treatment guidelines and making thoughtful decisions.

In the parts that follow, we will go over the significance of HIV testing and diagnosis during pregnancy, as well as the current treatment options and their ramifications. You will be more equipped to make educated decisions and actively engage in your healthcare journey as an HIV-positive pregnant woman if you grasp these factors.

1.4 The Importance of Pregnancy HIV Testing and Diagnosis

Timely testing and diagnosis are important steps in controlling HIV/AIDS during pregnancy. This section focuses on the significance of HIV testing for pregnant women, the value of early detection, and the various types of tests available.

The Importance of Early Testing

Early identification of HIV during pregnancy is critical for various reasons. To begin, knowing your HIV status allows you to receive proper medical care and actions to safeguard your health and prevent the infection from infecting your baby. Early ART initiation greatly reduces the likelihood of mother-to-child transmission and improves overall maternal and newborn health outcomes.

Second, early testing allows your healthcare experts to properly monitor your viral infection. Throughout your pregnancy, your load, CD4 count, and immunological function will be monitored. This information aids in treatment decisions and ensures that your healthcare team can give you the most effective and personalized care possible.

Tests available include antenatal screening and beyond.

For pregnant women, there are various types of HIV testing available, and the choice of test may vary depending on factors such as availability, local guidelines, and personal preferences. The following are the most common types of testing conducted during pregnancy:

Antenatal Screening: The initial step in HIV testing during pregnancy is usually antenatal screening. These tests are intended to identify HIV antibodies or antigens in the mother's blood. Enzyme immunoassay (EIA) and fast antibody testing are two common screening assays. If the test provides a positive result, more confirmatory testing is required.

Confirmatory Testing: If the prenatal screening test is positive, confirmatory tests are performed to confirm the existence of HIV infection. These techniques, such as the Western blot test or nucleic acid amplification tests (NAATs), selectively target HIV genetic material or antibodies to offer conclusive evidence of HIV infection.

Viral Load Testing: This test determines the level of HIV in the blood. This test is used to evaluate the efficacy of antiretroviral therapy (ART) and to monitor the level of virus suppression. During pregnancy, viral load testing is essential to check that your treatment strategy is working optimally to limit the risk of transmission.

CD4 Count: A CD4 count counts the number of CD4 cells in your blood, which is a measure of the health and function of your immune system. Monitoring your CD4 count during pregnancy allows your doctor to monitor your immunological function and make informed decisions regarding your care and treatment.

Informed Consent and Confidentiality: HIV testing during pregnancy requires confidentiality and informed permission. Healthcare practitioners are constrained by ethical and legal commitments to keep their HIV status private. You should be given clear information about the aim of the test, the implications of the results, and your rights as a patient before undergoing any testing.

Prioritizing HIV testing and diagnosis during pregnancy is a proactive step toward protecting your health and the health of your child. Early detection allows you to receive proper medical care and make educated decisions about your treatment choices and how to lower the risk of mother-to-child transmission.

In the next section, we will look at the available HIV/AIDS treatment choices during pregnancy and examine how they affect both the mother and the fetus. You may actively engage in your healthcare journey and make informed decisions that encourage the greatest potential outcomes for you and your baby if you understand these treatment alternatives.

1.5 Treatment Options and Their Consequences

When it comes to controlling HIV/AIDS during pregnancy, there are several therapeutic choices available to protect both the mother's and the baby's health. This section provides an overview of the therapy options available and their effects.

Benefits and Considerations of Antiretroviral Therapy (ART) During Pregnancy

Antiretroviral therapy (ART) is the cornerstone of HIV/AIDS treatment and is extremely efficient in inhibiting virus replication, lowering viral load in the body, and maintaining immune function. When it comes to pregnancy, ART is critical in preventing HIV transmission from mother to kid.

The following are some of the advantages of ART during pregnancy:

- Reducing the Risk of Transmission: Beginning ART during pregnancy, ideally before conception or as soon as possible, dramatically reduces the risk of transmission from mother to child. When used consistently and effectively, ART can lower the chance of transmission to less than 1%.

- ART not only reduces the probability of transmission, but it also improves the mother's overall health and immune function. It aids in the maintenance or improvement of CD4 cell levels, inhibits viral replication, and reduces the risk of opportunistic infections.

- Improving Infant Outcomes: By lowering the viral load in the mother, ART reduces the baby's chances of contracting HIV. This improves newborn health outcomes and enhances the likelihood of having an HIV-free baby.

Consider the following while considering ART during pregnancy:

Treatment Regimens: There are several types of ART regimens available, and the choice of regimen may be influenced by several factors, including individual health status, viral resistance patterns, and other considerations. Side effects are possible, as are pregnancy-specific issues. Your healthcare practitioner will collaborate with you to select the best ART regimen for your unique requirements.

Medication Safety: The safety of ART medications during pregnancy has been well-researched, and many of these medications are now regarded as safe for usage during pregnancy. However, some medications may have possible hazards, and the benefits of treatment are carefully balanced with any potential concerns. Your doctor will weigh the risks and advantages of various medications and advise you accordingly.

Adherence and monitoring: These are critical for the success of ART in suppressing the virus and minimizing the risk of transmission. To promote the best pregnancy outcomes, it is critical to assess viral load,

CD4 count, and drug adherence regularly. It is critical to collaborate with your healthcare team and follow their suggestions for medication monitoring and adherence.

Alternative Feeding Methods: Reducing Transmission Risk

Breastfeeding increases the likelihood of HIV transmission from an infected woman to her child. In areas where there are safe and inexpensive alternatives to nursing, it is widely suggested that HIV-positive moms forego breastfeeding entirely. Providing adequate alternate feeding choices, like formula or donor milk, helps to reduce the risk of transmission via breast milk.

It is crucial to note that breastfeeding advice may differ depending on individual circumstances, accessible resources, and regional guidelines. It is critical to talk with your healthcare practitioner to identify the best feeding method for your unique scenario.

Collaboration and monitoring of healthcare providers: Close collaboration with your healthcare practitioner is vital throughout your pregnancy. Regular prenatal checkups, as well as monitoring of viral load, CD4 count, and overall health, are required to ensure that your treatment plan is effective and tailored to your specific needs. Open communication with your healthcare team enables timely treatment modifications, the resolution of any concerns or side effects, and the optimization of health results for both you and your baby.

You may actively participate in your healthcare journey and make informed decisions alongside your healthcare practitioner if you understand the different treatment options, including ART and other feeding options. Treatment measures and attentive monitoring throughout pregnancy are critical in lowering the risk of mother-to-child transmission and promoting maternal and child health and well-being.

Chapter 2

Managing HIV/AIDS Pregnancy Health and Wellness

In this chapter, we will look at how to manage your health and wellness when pregnant and living with HIV/AIDS. We will provide direction and insights to assist you manage your particular journey, including self-care practices, mental well-being, nutrition, exercise, medication adherence, and preventive actions. We will also discuss crucial issues such as partner support, stigma, disclosure difficulties, and the responsibility of healthcare practitioners in delivering complete prenatal care and monitoring. You can improve your health and have a pleasant pregnant experience by taking a holistic approach to your well-being and utilizing the available support networks and services.

2.1 Understanding the Importance of Pregnancy Self-Care

Pregnancy brings about significant physical, emotional, and psychological changes. When you have HIV/AIDS, self-care becomes even more important to safeguard your health and the health of your kid. Taking care of yourself when pregnant entails putting your physical health, mental well-being, and general lifestyle first. In this section, we will discuss the significance of self-care during pregnancy and offer practical suggestions for incorporating it into your daily routine.

Physical Health: It is critical to maintain your physical health during pregnancy. This includes the following:

Adherence to your antiretroviral therapy (ART) regimen: Taking your medications as directed by your doctor aids in the management of your viral load and decreases the danger of transmission to your baby.

Prenatal check-ups regularly: Attending all of your scheduled Prenatal checkups allows your doctor to monitor your health, track the progression of your pregnancy, and make any required changes to your treatment plan.

Consuming nutritious foods: Such as fruits, vegetables, whole grains, lean proteins, and healthy fats, supplies necessary nutrients for both you and your kid. Consult a healthcare physician or a dietitian for specialized nutritional advice.

Drinking plenty of water: Taking lots of water throughout the day will help your general health and promote optimum hydration.

Getting enough rest: Because pregnancy can be physically taxing, it's critical to prioritize appropriate rest and sleep. Listen to your body and permit yourself to rest when necessary.

Emotional Well-Being: Pregnancy can cause a wide range of emotions, and it's critical to put your emotional well-being first. Here are some pointers:

- **Seek assistance:** Connect with support groups, counseling services, or HIV/AIDS organizations that provide emotional support to pregnant HIV/AIDS patients. Sharing your feelings and concerns with others who understand can be beneficial.

- **Stress management:** This involves engaging in activities that help you relax and lower stress, such as deep breathing exercises, meditation, mindfulness, or hobbies that you like.

- **Communicate with your healthcare team:** Communicate your emotions and concerns to your healthcare professional openly. If necessary, they can offer advice, resources, and referrals to additional support services.

Practices in Lifestyle and Self-Care

Engage in light exercise: Talk to your doctor about safe workouts to do while pregnant. Walking, prenatal yoga, and swimming can all be beneficial in circulation, stress management, and overall well-being.

Maintain good hygiene: By washing your hands regularly, maintaining dental hygiene, and adopting infection-prevention procedures.

Avoid dangerous substances: Avoid smoking, drinking alcohol, and using recreational drugs, as these can be harmful to your health and the health of your baby.

Prioritize fun: Make time for activities that bring you joy and relaxation, whether they be reading, listening to music, taking baths, or indulging in creative outlets. These exercises can aid in stress reduction and overall well-being.

Remember that self-care is not selfish; it is an essential component of preserving your and your baby's health. You can improve your physical health, mental well-being, and lifestyle choices by prioritizing them. Navigate HIV/AIDS pregnancy in a positive and empowered manner. Don't be afraid to seek advice and assistance from your healthcare practitioner and support networks during your pregnancy journey.

2.2 Emotional and Psychological Well-Being Navigation

Pregnancy can be a period of intense emotions and psychological upheavals, and it is critical to focus on your emotional and psychological well-being when living with HIV/AIDS. Managing your mental health throughout pregnancy is critical to having a great pregnant experience. In this section, we will look at ways to manage your emotional and psychological well-being while pregnant with HIV/AIDS.

- Seek Emotional Support: Speak with your physician: Your healthcare practitioner is an excellent source of support and advice. They can give you information, address your problems, and direct you to professional counseling or support groups.

- Make contact with support groups: Joining support groups for those living with HIV/AIDS during pregnancy can give a secure area to discuss experiences, worries, and ideas. Connecting with others who are going through similar things can help reduce feelings of loneliness. Share your sentiments and concerns with trusted family members, friends, or your spouse. Their understanding and support can create a calming and comfortable environment.

- Set aside time for self-care: Participate in activities that encourage relaxation, stress reduction, and self-care. This can include things like going on walks, practicing mindfulness or meditation, journaling, or participating in hobbies that offer you delight.

- Exercise self-compassion: Be gentle and understanding with yourself. It's important to permit yourself to rest, take pauses, and accept your feelings without judgment during pregnancy.

- Establish boundaries: Set firm limits to defend your emotional well-being. This may include saying no to additional commitments, prioritizing your needs, and articulating your limits to others.

Stress Management

- Determine your stressors: Recognize instances or conditions that add to your stress. This awareness enables you to devise strategies for minimizing or dealing with these triggers.

- Create stress-management strategies: Investigate stress-reduction techniques such as deep breathing exercises, progressive muscle relaxation, guided imagery, or engaging in relaxing and stress-reduction activities.

- Participate in frequent physical activity: Physical activity has been shown to improve mental health and reduce stress. Consult your healthcare practitioner about safe exercises to do while pregnant.

- Therapy or counseling: Consider getting professional counseling or therapy if you are suffering substantial emotional pain or are difficult to manage. Mental health specialists with previous work experience with people living with HIV/AIDS, can get advice, coping tactics, and support throughout your pregnancy experience.

- Psychiatric care: Medication or psychiatric help may be required in some circumstances to manage mental health issues such as depression or anxiety. Discuss the potential advantages and hazards of medication during pregnancy with your healthcare professional.

- Discover more about HIV/AIDS and pregnancy: Educating yourself about the medical issues of HIV/AIDS during pregnancy can help reduce worry and enable you to make educated decisions about your own and your baby's health. Request credible resources from your healthcare physician or attend HIV/AIDS-specific educational courses.

- Keep in mind that emotional well-being is a journey, and it is natural to feel a variety of emotions during pregnancy.

You can better navigate the emotional and psychological elements of HIV/AIDS pregnancy by obtaining support, practicing self-care, controlling stress, seeking professional help when necessary, and educating yourself. Your mental health is important, and prioritizing it helps you have a happier and more happy pregnant experience.

2.3 Nutrition and Diet Factors to Consider for a Healthy Pregnancy

A nutritious and balanced diet is vital during pregnancy, especially if you have HIV/AIDS. Proper eating benefits your general health, stimulates your immune system, and supplies the nutrients required for your baby's development. This section will go over crucial nutrition and food factors for a safe HIV/AIDS pregnancy.

Consume a Wide Range of Nutrient-Dense Foods

- **Vegetables and fruits:** Include a wide variety of fruits and vegetables in your diet to guarantee adequate vitamin, mineral, and antioxidant intake. To maximize nutrient consumption, aim for at least five servings each day and choose colorful selections.

- **Choose whole grain foods:** Such as whole wheat bread, brown rice, and oats. These offer fiber, B vitamins, and other minerals that are all important. Poultry, fish, eggs, lentils, and tofu are examples of lean protein sources. These provide essential elements such as iron and folate.

- **Healthy Fats:** Include healthy fats from avocados, nuts, seeds, and olive oil. These lipids are necessary for prenatal brain development as well as overall wellness.

- **Dairy or Dairy Substitutes**: To achieve enough calcium intake, consume dairy products or acceptable alternatives such as fortified plant-based pints of milk.

Adequate protein and iron consumption

- **Protein:** Make sure you get enough protein for your baby's growth and development. Lean meats, chicken, fish, beans, dairy products, and tofu are all good sources.

- **Iron**: This is necessary for the synthesis of red blood cells and the transfer of oxygen. Include iron-rich meals such as lean meats, poultry, fish, leafy greens, legumes, and fortified cereals into your diet. To improve iron absorption, consume vitamin C-rich meals (such as citrus fruits) alongside iron-rich foods.

- Focus on Hydration: To stay hydrated, drink plenty of water throughout the day. Hydration is important for overall health, digestion, and nutrition absorption.

Food Safety Procedures

Use proper food hygiene and safety precautions: Wash your hands before preparing or eating food, completely prepare meat, and avoid cross-contamination of raw and cooked meals.

Certain foods should be avoided: Some foods are more prone to contamination and should be avoided when pregnant. Unpasteurized dairy products, raw or undercooked seafood, deli meats, and certain types of fish with high mercury levels are examples.

Consult a Medical Professional or a Nutritionist

Each person's nutritional requirements are distinct, consult your healthcare practitioner or a qualified dietitian to create a customized dietary plan that takes your HIV status and any other special needs into account.

Nutrition with Antiretroviral Therapy (ART)

Work with your doctor to ensure that your antiretroviral medication (ART) regimen and dietary choices are in sync. Some drugs may necessitate special dietary considerations or timing of meal consumption.

Vitamins for Pregnancy

Prenatal vitamins should be taken as directed by your healthcare professional. Prenatal vitamins can help cover nutritional shortages and guarantee proper vitamin and mineral consumption.

Remember that an appropriate diet is essential for your health as well as your baby's optimal development. By eating a diverse and nutrient-dense diet, staying hydrated, practicing proper food handling, and obtaining medical advice from Professionals, you can help your well-being during an HIV/AIDS pregnancy.

2.4 Guidelines for Physical Fitness and Exercise

Staying physically active throughout pregnancy is good for your general health as well as the health of your kid. It is critical to prioritize physical fitness and exercise safely when living with HIV/AIDS. In this section, we will look at the rules and considerations for being physically active while pregnant with HIV/AIDS.

- Consult Your Healthcare Practitioner: Before beginning or continuing an exercise routine while pregnant, consult your healthcare practitioner. They can examine your health status, provide specific recommendations, and answer any concerns you may have about your HIV/AIDS condition.

Select Appropriate Activities

- **Choose low-impact exercises:** Choose activities that are easy on your joints and reduce your risk of injury. Walking, swimming, stationary cycling, and prenatal yoga are among examples as well as low-impact exercises.
- **Exercises should be modified as needed:** Adapt your workouts to your changing physique and energy levels. Choose a slower pace, reduce the intensity, or use props or modifications suggested by prenatal exercise instructors, for example.
- **Avoid high-impact activities such as:** Avoid activities that require jumping, quick movements, or a high risk of falling or impact to the abdomen, as these can endanger your and your baby's safety.

Precautions for Safety

- **Warm-up and cool-down periods:** Warm up your muscles and gradually increase your heart rate before beginning any exercise activity. After that, stretch your muscles and gradually drop your heart rate.
- **Keep hydrated:** To avoid dehydration, drink plenty of water before, during, and after exercise.

- **Pay attention to your body:** Pay attention to how you feel when exercising. Stop exercising and visit your healthcare practitioner if you have pain, dizziness, shortness of breath, or any other discomfort.
- **Prevent overheating:** Avoid exercising in hot and humid weather. Consider exercising in well-ventilated settings or inside.
- **Wear proper attire:** Choose exercise-appropriate apparel that is loose-fitting, breathable, and comfortable, as well as supportive footwear.
- **Exercises for the Pelvic Floor:** Incorporate Kegel exercises, commonly known as pelvic floor exercises, into your routine. These exercises can help avoid urine incontinence during and after pregnancy by strengthening the muscles that support the pelvic organs.
- **Gradual Development:** If you were physically active before becoming pregnant, you may be able to continue with your exercise program with some modifications. However, it is critical to pay attention to your body and gradually adapt to pregnancy's shifting needs. Start with easy activities and progressively increase duration and intensity as prescribed by your healthcare practitioner if you were not physically active before pregnancy.
- **Considerations for ART:** whether you are on antiretroviral therapy (ART), see your healthcare physician to see whether any special exercise precautions are required based on your medication regimen.
- **Discomforts Associated with Pregnancy:** Pregnancy might cause some discomfort, such as back pain or joint pain. If you feel any discomfort when exercising, adapt the activity or attempt a different workout that is more pleasant for you.

Keep in mind that every pregnancy is different, and what works for one person may not work for another. It is critical to listen to your body and seek advice from your healthcare practitioner and adjust your workout plan as appropriate. Maintaining physical fitness throughout HIV/AIDS pregnancy might help you improve your general health, manage stress, and even improve your labor and delivery experience.

2.5 Medication Management and Treatment Adherence

Managing medications and following the approved treatment regimen is critical for your health and the prevention of mother-to-child transmission when living with HIV/AIDS during pregnancy. We will explore ways for efficiently managing your medications and maintaining treatment adherence during pregnancy in this section.

Maintain Open and Honest Communication with Your Healthcare Provider: Maintain open and honest communication with your healthcare provider about your HIV/AIDS treatment plan and any issues or challenges you may experience. They can offer advice, answer questions, and offer support throughout your pregnancy.

Recognize Your Medications

Learn about the medications you're taking, including their intended use, dosages, and potential side effects. This knowledge will enable you to make informed decisions about your treatment and actively engage in it.

Follow the suggested Treatment Plan

Follow the medication schedule suggested by your healthcare professional. Take your drugs at the appropriate times and in the appropriate doses. If necessary, set reminders or alarms to help you remember.

Address Potential Side Effects

Certain drugs may produce nausea, tiredness, or gastrointestinal pain. Discuss this with your healthcare practitioner if you develop side effects that interfere with your ability to take your prescriptions. They may be able to recommend alternative medications or ways of dealing with adverse effects.

Involve Your Support Network

Inform your partner, family members, or close friends about your treatment plan and the importance of sticking to it. Seek their help and support in ensuring that you take your prescriptions exactly as prescribed, especially if you are tired or have forgotten something.

Properly organize and store medications

Organize your prescriptions in a way that works best for you. To guarantee that you have the right prescriptions at the right time, use pill organizers or other solutions. Keep your prescriptions in a cool, dry area, away from direct sunlight, and out of children's reach.

Considerations for Travel

If you want to travel throughout your pregnancy, be sure you have an adequate supply of drugs. To avoid problems with lost or delayed luggage, keep prescriptions in your carry-on bag. Consult your healthcare practitioner about modifying your medication schedule if you are traveling to a different time zone.

Seek Help and Resources

Contact HIV/AIDS organizations, support groups, or other organizations. These resources can provide vital information, encouragement, and support from people who have faced similar difficulties.

Take Care of Your Mental Health

Treatment adherence is heavily influenced by mental health. Seek help from a mental health expert if you are suffering from depression, anxiety, or other mental health issues. They can assist you in developing coping techniques and providing the essential support to ensure that you adhere to your treatment plan.

Monitoring and follow-up regularly

Attend all prenatal appointments and laboratory testing as scheduled to monitor your HIV status and the success of your therapy. Regular monitoring allows your healthcare provider to make any required adjustments to your drug regimen and guarantee your and your baby's health and well-being.

Remember to keep track of your meds

Proper adherence to treatment is critical for your health and the avoidance of mother-to-child transmission. You may maximize the benefits of your medicine and ensure a healthy pregnancy with HIV/AIDS by actively participating in your treatment plan, finding assistance, and addressing any obstacles or concerns.

2.6 Opportunistic Infections and Their Complications

When living with HIV/AIDS throughout pregnancy, avoiding opportunistic infections and complications is critical for your health and the health of your baby. In this section, we will go through measures for preventing opportunistic infections and managing potential complications during HIV/AIDS pregnancy.

Adherence to Antiretroviral Therapy (ART)

Strictly follow your antiretroviral therapy (ART) schedule. ART decreases viral replication, strengthens your immune system, and minimizes your risk of opportunistic infections. Maintain regular follow-up appointments and take your prescriptions as instructed by your healthcare professional.

Attend Prenatal Care Visits regularly

Attend all planned prenatal care visits. These appointments allow your doctor to keep an eye on your health, test your immune system, and detect any potential issues or infections at an early stage. Adhere to the HIV/AIDS-specific prenatal care guidelines.

Keep a Healthy Lifestyle

To strengthen your immune system and overall health, eat a nutritious and balanced diet. Include immune-boosting foods in your diet, such as fruits, vegetables, whole grains, lean meats, and healthy fats.

- To improve your immune function, reduce stress, and maintain general well-being, engage in regular physical activity as directed by your healthcare physician.
- To boost your immune system and overall health, get enough rest and practice excellent sleep hygiene.

Maintain Good Hygiene

Wash your hands with soap and water frequently, especially before preparing or eating food, using the restroom, or being in public places. Hand cleanliness is important in preventing the spread of diseases.

Avoid direct touch with individuals suffering from active illnesses, particularly respiratory diseases. Wear a mask or adopt social distancing if necessary to limit the danger of exposure.

Immunizations: Follow your healthcare provider's recommendations for immunizations. Influenza and pneumococcal immunizations, for example, can help prevent common infections and consequences.

Consult your doctor about which immunizations are safe and recommended during pregnancy.

Sexually Transmitted Infections (STIs) Prevention

Use barrier techniques, such as condoms, correctly and consistently during sexual activity to practice safe sex. This reduces the danger of developing sexually transmitted illnesses, which can weaken the immune system even further.

Food and Water Infection Prevention

Ensure proper food safety practices, such as properly washing fruits and vegetables and cooking food to the proper temperature as well as avoiding eating raw or undercooked meats or seafood.

Drink only clean, safe water. If the quality of tap water worries you, go with bottled or filtered water.

Stress Management

Chronic stress can compromise the immune system. Deep breathing exercises, meditation, yoga, or indulging in things that offer you joy and relaxation are all effective stress management approaches.

Seek Immediate Medical Attention

Seek medical assistance right away if you have any symptoms of infection or problems, such as fever, prolonged cough, diarrhea, or unusual vaginal discharge. Early detection and treatment can help prevent infections or problems from progressing.

Communicate with Your Medical Professional

Maintain open and honest contact with your healthcare practitioner about any health concerns, symptoms, or changes. They may be able to supply appropriate guidance, answer your concerns, and personalize your care to manage any potential dangers.

Remember that prevention is essential in controlling opportunistic infections and problems associated with HIV/AIDS during pregnancy. You can reduce the risk of opportunistic infections and complications and promote a healthier pregnancy for both you and your baby by sticking to your ART regimen, attending regular prenatal care visits, maintaining a healthy lifestyle, practicing good hygiene, receiving recommended vaccinations, preventing STIs, managing stress, and seeking prompt medical attention.

2.7 HIV/AIDS and Pregnancy Support Systems and Resources

Navigating pregnancy with HIV/AIDS can be difficult, but you don't have to go through it alone. Throughout your journey, there are many support systems and services available to provide aid, guidance, and emotional support. In this section, we will look at several helpful support systems and tools that can assist you during your HIV/AIDS pregnancy.

Healthcare Providers: Your healthcare team, which includes obstetricians, gynecologists, and infectious disease specialists, is critical to managing your HIV/AIDS pregnancy. They can give you medical advice, check your health, change treatment programs, and answer any questions or concerns you may have.

Organizations working on HIV/AIDS: Many organizations specialize in assisting those living with HIV/AIDS. These organizations provide information, educational materials, support groups, and other services, as well as pregnancy and HIV/AIDS counseling services. Local HIV/AIDS service organizations, national organizations such as the HIV Medicine Association, and worldwide organizations such as UNAIDS are examples.

Peer Support Organizations: Connecting with other people who have had or are experiencing HIV/AIDS pregnancies can provide vital support and understanding. Look for local or online support groups where you can share your experiences, exchange information, and get encouragement from people who understand your position.

Professionals in Mental Health: During pregnancy, your mental health is extremely important to your overall well-being. Seeking the help of a mental health expert, such as a counselor, therapist, or psychologist, can help you address any emotional issues, manage stress, and build coping techniques tailored to your situation.

Social Workers: Social workers can help you in a variety of ways, handling different elements of your pregnancy journey, such as obtaining healthcare, managing financial worries, understanding your rights and benefits, and connecting you with community resources. They can also offer emotional support and assist in the coordination of your care.

Case Managers: Case managers are trained professionals who coordinate care for people living with HIV/AIDS. Throughout your pregnancy, they can assist you in obtaining medical and social resources, ensuring treatment adherence, providing education, and advocating for your needs.

Resources and information available online

- There are various trustworthy websites and online platforms that provide pregnancy and HIV/AIDS-related information, educational materials, and tools. Examples include the ***websites of the Centers for Disease Control and Prevention (CDC)***, the ***World Health Organization (WHO), and HIV/AIDS-focused websites such as TheBody.com***.

- **Books and educational materials:** and literature on HIV/AIDS pregnancy can provide helpful insights, information, and reassurance. Look for books published by healthcare experts or people who have firsthand knowledge of HIV/AIDS during pregnancy. These resources can provide useful advice, emotional support, and up-to-date information.

Programs for the Local Community

Investigate local community initiatives, such as support groups, counseling services, or prenatal education classes, that may be provided expressly for pregnant HIV/AIDS patients. These programs can offer additional assistance, knowledge, and a sense of belonging.

Friends and family

Seek emotional support and understanding from your loved ones. Inform them about your circumstances, educate them about HIV/AIDS, and talk about how they can support you throughout your pregnancy.

Remember that seeking out help is a good thing, it is a sign of strength, and there are tools available to help you during your HIV/AIDS pregnancy. These support systems and resources can provide guidance, information, emotional support, and a sense of community as you navigate your unique journey, whether through healthcare providers, organizations, support groups, mental health professionals, online resources, or your support network.

2.8 Overcoming Stigma and Disclosure Obstacles

Living with HIV/AIDS during pregnancy might be accompanied by stigma and disclosure difficulties. Addressing these concerns is critical for promoting emotional well-being and creating a supportive workplace. In this section, we will cover ways to deal with stigma and overcome obstacles associated with HIV/AIDS disclosure during pregnancy.

Educate Yourself: Gain a thorough understanding of HIV/AIDS to dispel any misunderstandings or misconceptions. Learn about the facts, transmission methods, treatment options, and recent advances in HIV/AIDS care. This understanding will enable you to handle stigma confidently and engage in educated debates.

Seek Assistance: Connect with support groups or counseling programs intended exclusively for people living with HIV/AIDS. These areas provide a secure and understanding environment, individuals who have had similar issues can share their stories, offer advice, and provide emotional support.

Establish open and honest conversations with your healthcare physician, partner, and other trustworthy people in your life. Discuss your concerns, fears, and disclosure-related experiences. They can offer advice, support, and assistance in negotiating these difficulties.

- **Create a Supportive Network**

Surround yourself with people who understand and accept you, such as family, friends, or support groups. These people can offer emotional support, fight stigma, and help you make decisions about disclosure.

Considerations for Disclosure

Disclosure is a personal choice, and you have the freedom to select who you tell about your HIV/AIDS status. Consider the potential benefits carefully and the hazards of disclosing in different circumstances, such as your healthcare, relationships, and workplace.

- Consider your level of comfort, the trustworthiness of the people involved, and the potential impact of disclosure on your well-being.
- Remember that disclosure does not have to be all or nothing. You have the option of disclosing selectively, only to those who need to know or with whom you feel comfortable sharing.

Self-Care and Coping Techniques

Self-care activities that improve emotional well-being, such as meditation, mindfulness, writing, or hobbies, should be practiced. These techniques can help you manage stress, develop resilience, and boost your self-esteem. Create coping mechanisms to deal with stigma, such as educating people, disputing misunderstandings, and seeking help when necessary. Participating in advocacy activities may also enable you to feel more empowered, and, on a larger scale, less stigmatized.

Know Your Rights: Learn about the legal protections and rights available to those living with HIV/AIDS in your country or region. Understanding your rights can offer you a sense of empowerment and assist you in dealing with any discrimination or stigma-related issues that may emerge.

Managing Internalized Stigma: Internalized stigma refers to unfavorable thoughts and feelings that people may internalize as a result of societal stigma. Recognize and question any self-stigmatizing thoughts or beliefs that occur. Engage in self-compassion and remind yourself that being HIV/AIDS positive does not determine your worth or ability as a person.

Educate Others: Consider educating individuals close to you about HIV/AIDS, such as family, friends, or coworkers, to dispel misunderstandings and misconceptions. Providing accurate information might be beneficial, reduce stigma and foster a more accepting environment. Participate in advocacy initiatives to enhance HIV/AIDS awareness, battle stigma, and promote access to healthcare and support services. You may help to create a more inclusive and understanding society by lobbying for change.

Remember that dealing with stigma and disclosure issues is a personal journey, and it is critical to prioritize your mental well-being and self-care throughout. You may combat stigma by obtaining help, engaging in open communication, creating coping techniques, and pushing for change.

2.9 Partner Support and Participation in the Pregnancy Journey

Having your partner's support during your HIV/AIDS pregnancy can make a huge difference in your general well-being and the successful management of your illness. In this section, we will discuss the significance of partner support and involvement, as well as suggestions for fostering a supportive partnership during your pregnancy.

Open and Honest Communication: Establish an open and honest communication foundation with your relationship. Talk about your feelings, fears, and needs concerning your HIV/AIDS diagnosis and pregnancy. Encourage your partner to express their feelings and views as well. This will establish a safe environment for comprehension and assistance. Encourage your partner to learn about HIV/AIDS, including transmission, treatment, and management, during their pregnancy. This information will assist them in better understanding your situation and the actions needed in managing your and your baby's health.

Attending Your Medical Appointments

Invite your partner to accompany you to prenatal care appointments. This allows them to actively engage in your healthcare journey, ask questions, and develop a better awareness of the medical elements of HIV/AIDS management while pregnant.

Emotional Assistance: Tell your partner about your emotional experiences and concerns. Inform them of how their emotional support can benefit their well-being. Encourage them to offer a listening ear, words of support, and empathy throughout the pregnancy.

Assistance with Medication Adherence: Ask your spouse to help you remember to take your antiretroviral pills regularly. They can play an important role in assisting you to adhere to your medication schedule, which is essential for controlling HIV/AIDS throughout pregnancy.

Promoting Healthy Lifestyle Options: Participate in healthy lifestyle choices as a family. Encourage each other to eat a balanced diet, exercise regularly, and engage in stress-relieving activities. You may improve your general well-being by encouraging each other to make healthy choices.

Preparing for Parenthood and Birth: Attend birthing or parenting classes together. These lectures teach important information on labor and delivery, baby care, and HIV/AIDS considerations throughout pregnancy. Participating as a pair will make you both feel more prepared and involved in your baby's impending arrival.

Addressing Concerns and Fears: Make a comfortable environment for your spouse to discuss their anxieties as well as concerns regarding HIV/AIDS and the pregnancy path. Pay close attention, affirm their emotions, and reassure them. You can work together to address any concerns and develop solutions.

Partner Support Networks: Encourage your partner to seek their own support network or counseling programs designed specifically for partners of HIV/AIDS patients. Connecting with individuals who have gone through similar things might provide them with extra support and understanding.

Milestone & Achievement Recognition: Take time to celebrate your pregnancy's milestones and accomplishments. This can include receiving positive medical reports, establishing viral suppression, or meeting critical pregnancy milestones. Recognize and appreciate your partner's contribution to your achievement.

Remember that your partner's support and involvement are invaluable resources during your HIV/AIDS pregnancy. By encouraging open communication, you can enhance your partnership and manage the pregnancy journey together by encouraging education, providing emotional support, and incorporating them into your medical treatment.

2.10 Prenatal Care and Consistent Monitoring

Prenatal care and regular monitoring are critical components of managing your HIV/AIDS health during pregnancy. In this section, we will discuss the significance of prenatal care and regular monitoring, as well as provide an overview of what to expect throughout these critical stages of your pregnancy.

The Importance of Prenatal Care: Prenatal care is critical to the health of both you and your baby. Regular check-ups with your healthcare practitioner enable health monitoring, HIV/AIDS management, and the detection and prevention of any potential consequences.

Developing a Relationship of Trust with Your Healthcare Provider: It is critical to have a trusting relationship with your healthcare practitioner. Select an HIV/AIDS specialist provider that has prior expertise in handling pregnancies in people with the illness. This will guarantee that you get the finest treatment and support possible during your pregnancy.

First Prenatal Visit

Your healthcare practitioner will do a comprehensive evaluation of your health during your first prenatal visit, including a thorough medical history review, physical examination, and laboratory tests. They will go over your HIV/AIDS diagnosis, treatment plan, and any changes that may be required during pregnancy.

Continued Prenatal Visits

Subsequent prenatal checkups are normally scheduled every 4-6 weeks during the early stages of pregnancy, increasing in frequency as your due date approaches. During these appointments, your overall health will be monitored, the progression of your pregnancy will be tracked, and the status of your HIV/AIDS care will be assessed.

Keeping an Eye on the Viral Load: During pregnancy, it is critical to have your viral load (the quantity of HIV in your blood) checked regularly. Keeping your viral load low with antiretroviral medication (ART) is critical for reducing the risk of HIV transmission from mother to child.

Monitoring of CD4 Cell Count: The CD4 cell count, a measure of the immune system's health, is examined during pregnancy. This aids in determining the impact of HIV/AIDS on your immune system and the best course of treatment.

Additional Laboratory Tests: Your healthcare professional may suggest additional laboratory tests to evaluate your overall health and your baby's well-being. Complete blood counts, liver function tests, kidney function testing, and tests for other sexually transmitted infections (STIs) may be included.

Ultrasounds and Fetal Monitoring: Ultrasounds are commonly used during pregnancy, to monitor your baby's growth and development. Your healthcare professional may also propose additional ultrasounds to assess the baby's well-being and potential issues. Non-stress tests or biophysical profiles, for example, may be used to monitor your baby's health and well-being during pregnancy.

Treatment Modifications: To maximize the management of your HIV/AIDS, your healthcare professional may need to make changes to your antiretroviral therapy regimen during pregnancy. To avoid mother-to-child transmission, drugs may be changed, dosages adjusted, or extra medications added.

Making Decisions Together: Throughout the prenatal care and monitoring process, your healthcare professional will involve you in the treatment plan and HIV/AIDS management decisions. Collaborative decision-making guarantees that your individual wants and preferences are taken into account.

Remember that prenatal care and regular monitoring are critical for controlling your health and maintaining the safety of both you and your baby during an HIV/AIDS pregnancy. You can take proactive steps toward a healthy pregnancy and the prevention of HIV transmission from mother to child by attending regular prenatal visits, monitoring your viral load and CD4 cell count, undergoing necessary laboratory tests and ultrasounds, and actively participating in decision-making.

2.11 Positive Mental Health Promotion and Coping Strategies

Maintaining excellent mental health and using appropriate coping methods are critical parts of managing an HIV/AIDS pregnancy. In this section, we will discuss the significance of promoting positive mental health and offer solutions for dealing with emotional issues that may arise during this journey.

Recognize and validate your feelings throughout your pregnancy journey. It is common to feel a variety of emotions, such as dread, anxiety, grief, or uncertainty. Allow yourself to openly express your emotions and seek help from trusted individuals or support groups.

Seek Professional Help: Consider counseling or therapy with a mental health professional who has experience working with people living with HIV/AIDS. Professional assistance can establish a secure environment.

Create a Support System: Surround yourself with a support network of people who can offer emotional support, encouragement, and understanding. This network could consist of your partner, family, friends, or support groups. Connect with these people regularly to share your experiences and seek advice.

Self-care is essential: Make self-care activities that boost your overall well-being a priority. Engage in enjoyable activities such as reading, listening to music, practicing mindfulness or meditation, or participating in hobbies. Taking care of your physical, emotional, and spiritual needs will help you achieve better mental health.

Communicate with your companion: Maintain open and honest communication about your emotional well-being with your partner. Inform them of your concerns, fears, and needs, and urge them to do the same. Throughout the pregnancy, you can provide each other with support, understanding, and reassurance.

Prepare Yourself: Educate yourself on HIV/AIDS, pregnancy, and the services and support systems that are accessible. Knowledge enables you to make informed decisions, dispel myths, and advocate for your well-being. Keep up to date on advances in HIV/AIDS management and seek out credible sources of information.

Set reasonable expectations: Set reasonable goals for yourself during your pregnancy. Recognize that ups and downs are normal and that you may experience them. Be gentle with yourself, practice self-compassion, and realize that you are doing your best.

Create Coping Strategies: Determine and implement the coping strategies that are most effective for you. Deep breathing exercises, journaling, relaxation techniques, physical activity, and participation in support groups are examples of such activities. Experiment with different tactics to see what works best for you in terms of stress management and mental health.

Dispel Stigma and Discrimination: Speak out against HIV/AIDS stigma and discrimination. Educate people, dispel myths, and push for a more accepting and understanding society. As an advocate, you may help to reduce the stigma associated with HIV/AIDS and promote positive mental health.

Celebrate Significant Milestones and Achievements: Celebrate your accomplishments and milestones throughout your path of pregnancy. Recognize and value your perseverance, courage, and capacity to manage your HIV/AIDS while fostering a new life. Celebrating these occasions can increase your self-esteem and encourage good mental health. Remember that encouraging positive mental health and using appropriate coping skills are critical for your overall well-being during an HIV/AIDS pregnancy. You may negotiate the emotional hurdles and appreciate the wonderful moments of this journey by recognizing and expressing your emotions, getting help, practicing self-care, and educating yourself.

2.12 Pregnancy and Family Planning Options for HIV-Infected People

Pregnancy and family planning options for people living with HIV/AIDS must be carefully considered to ensure the health and well-being of both the parent and the child. In this section, we will address the significance of pregnancy planning, the numerous family planning choices accessible to HIV-positive people, and how to make informed decisions about motherhood.

Pregnancy Planning: Pregnancy planning is critical for those living with HIV/AIDS to reduce the risk of transferring the virus to their partners and unborn child. Planning allows for the best possible care of the disease, as well as access to required medical measures and supports to ensure a successful pregnancy and birth.

Consultation with a Healthcare Professional: It is essential to see your doctor before attempting to become pregnant. It is critical to contact a healthcare physician who has experience managing HIV/AIDS and reproductive health. They can offer advice, examine your health status, alter prescriptions as needed, and make recommendations based on your specific circumstances.

Antiretroviral medication (ART) and Viral Suppression: Before attempting pregnancy, it is critical to achieve and maintain viral suppression with adequate antiretroviral medication (ART). This lessens the chance of viral transmission to your partner and dramatically reduces the risk of mother-to-child transmission during pregnancy and childbirth.

Conception choices: If you have an HIV-negative or HIV-positive partner, there are several conception choices available to reduce the risk of transmission. These include timed intercourse during your most fertile period, intrauterine insemination (IUI) with processed sperm, and in vitro fertilization (IVF) with pre-implantation genetic testing used to select HIV-negative embryos.

Preconception Care: Preconception care is critical for optimizing your health before getting pregnant. Addressing any underlying medical concerns, ensuring vaccines are up to date, monitoring drug regimens, and assessing general reproductive health are all part of this process.

Family Planning Alternatives: There are numerous family planning options if pregnancy is not desired or recommended. Barrier methods (such as condoms), hormonal methods (such as birth control tablets or patches), intrauterine devices (IUDs), contraceptive implants, or sterilization operations are examples of such approaches. Discuss these possibilities with your healthcare practitioner to determine which option is best for you.

Considerations for HIV-Infected Women: Additional considerations for HIV-positive women include potential interactions between antiretroviral drugs and contraception techniques. Certain contraceptives are contraindicated; therefore, it is critical to consult with your healthcare professional to determine the best alternative.

Pregnancy Contraception: It is critical to continue using effective contraception until you and your healthcare physician conclude that it is safe to attempt pregnancy. This aids in the prevention of unplanned pregnancies and ensures that you are fully prepared for a healthy pregnancy.

Counseling and assistance: Seek advice from healthcare professionals, support groups, and counseling programs specializing in HIV/AIDS and reproductive health throughout the decision-making process. These tools can help you negotiate the intricacies of pregnancy and family planning by providing guidance, addressing concerns, and providing emotional support.

Decisions Reconsidered: It is critical to reevaluate your pregnancy decisions when your circumstances change or new information becomes available. Consult with your healthcare physician regularly to discuss any changes in HIV management and reproductive health alternatives.

Remember that pregnancy and family planning options for HIV-positive people require serious thought and consultation with healthcare specialists. You can make informed decisions that emphasize your health and the well-being of your partner and possible child by working closely with your healthcare practitioner, engaging in preconception care, and investigating appropriate family planning alternatives.

2.13 Education and Counseling on Sexual and Reproductive Health

Sexual and reproductive health education and counseling are critical components of comprehensive care for HIV/AIDS patients who are thinking about getting pregnant or navigating their reproductive health. In this section, we will discuss the significance of sexual and reproductive health education, as well as the advantages of counseling in promoting informed decision-making and general well-being.

Importance of Sexual and Reproductive Health Education: Sexual and reproductive health education is critical for people living with HIV/AIDS to make educated sexual and reproductive health decisions. It informs readers on the risks of transmission, preventative strategies, fertility alternatives, and available support resources.

Risks of Transmission and Prevention

Understanding the risks of HIV transmission and the various preventative measures is critical. Sexual and reproductive health education can teach people about safe sexual behaviors, such as using condoms consistently and correctly, the significance of sticking to antiretroviral therapy (ART), and how to reduce the risk of transmission to partners.

Family Planning and Fertility Options

Individuals living with HIV/AIDS can benefit from sexual and reproductive health education to learn about fertility alternatives and family planning. This contains debates about different techniques of conception, assisted reproductive technologies, contraception methods, and the potential influence of HIV on fertility.

Safer Methods of Conception

Through sexual and reproductive health education, safer conception techniques such as timed intercourse, Prep for the HIV-negative partner, and viral suppression through ART can be explored. These measures help to reduce the chance of transmission while attempting to conceive.

Prenatal Care and Pregnancy Planning: Sexual Reproductive health education can help with pregnancy planning, preconception care, and the necessity of optimizing general health before trying for a baby.

Addressing underlying medical issues, managing medications, and fostering a healthy lifestyle are all part of this.

Education and counseling: Can help with the difficulties of disclosing and communicating about HIV status with partners, family members, and healthcare providers. It offers ways for effectively navigating these talks and highlights the value of open and honest communication.

Psychosocial Support: Sexual and reproductive health education and counseling can provide psychosocial support to HIV/AIDS patients. It aids in the treatment of emotional issues, stigma, and the impact of HIV on sexual and reproductive decisions. Self-esteem, resilience, and overall well-being can all benefit from supportive therapy.

Access to Resources and Assistance: Sexual and reproductive individuals are connected to accessible services and support networks through reproductive health education. Referrals to specialized healthcare providers, HIV/AIDS clinics, support groups, and counseling services are all part of this. The availability of these resources ensures that women receive complete treatment and support throughout their reproductive health journey.

Making Informed Decisions: Individuals can make informed decisions about their sexual and reproductive health with the help of education and counseling. They give a forum for people to discuss their personal values, desires, and concerns while also taking into account the medical, emotional, and social elements of HIV/AIDS and reproductive choices.

Continuous Support and Follow-Up: Sexual and reproductive health education and counseling should be a continuous process with continuing support and follow-up. Regular meetings can address shifting requirements, provide research and advancement updates, and allow individuals to reexamine their reproductive health goals as well as ideas.

Remember that sexual and reproductive health education and counseling are critical for HIV/AIDS patients. Individuals can navigate their reproductive health with confidence and make choices that match their values, well-being, and intended outcomes by receiving knowledge, getting assistance, and engaging in informed decision-making.

2.14 Managing Antiretroviral Therapy (ART) Potential Side Effects

Antiretroviral therapy (ART) is a cornerstone of HIV/AIDS management, aiding in virus suppression and overall wellness. However, ART, like any drug, has the possibility of negative effects. In this part, we will address common ART side effects and ways for effectively controlling them.

Understanding Common Adverse Effects: Become acquainted with the potential adverse effects of the antiretroviral drugs you are taking. Nausea, diarrhea, lethargy, headache, rash, or changes in body fat distribution are common side effects. Being aware of these side effects might assist you in proactively identifying and managing them.

Communication with the Healthcare Provider: Maintain open communication with your healthcare practitioner about any adverse effects. Inform them of the nature, severity, and duration of the symptoms. This allows them to assess the situation and, if necessary, make changes to your prescription plan.

Medication Schedule Adherence: It is critical to stick to your medication schedule. Skipping or changing dosages can result in diminished effectiveness and treatment failure. Taking your medicine as advised by your healthcare professional reduces the chance of side effects while increasing the therapeutic advantages of ART.

Considerations for Timing and Food: Some antiretroviral drugs must be taken with food, while others should be taken on an empty stomach. Follow your healthcare provider's particular advice regarding timing and food requirements. This can help with gastrointestinal side symptoms like nausea and diarrhea.

Supportive Care for Gastrointestinal Disorders and Side Effects: There are numerous supportive measures you can take if you have gastrointestinal side effects. These include staying hydrated by drinking enough fluids, eating small, frequent meals, avoiding hot or oily foods, and including fiber-rich foods in your diet. Over-the-counter drugs such as anti-nausea or antidiarrheal pills may also provide brief relief. Fatigue and headaches are common side effects of certain antiretroviral medicines. Rest, a regular sleep routine, relaxation techniques, and stress management can all assist to reduce these symptoms. If your headaches persist or worsen, see your doctor for further examination and treatment.

Skin Rash and Hypersensitivity Reactions: Certain antiretroviral drugs can cause skin rash or hypersensitivity reactions. It is critical to get medical attention if you develop a rash, they can analyze the severity of the rash and determine whether prescription changes or extra treatment are required.

Counseling and Psychological Support: Managing potential ART side effects might have emotional and psychological consequences. To address any fears or anxiety, seek help from healthcare professionals, counseling services, or support groups. Psychological assistance can help patients cope with side effects, improve drug adherence, and promote general well-being.

Monitoring and laboratory tests regularly: Regular health monitoring and laboratory tests are critical components of HIV/AIDS care. These tests aid in determining the efficacy of your drug, monitoring any adverse effects, and assessing your overall health. Following the prescribed monitoring plan enables early discovery and control of any problems.

Medication Regimen Modifications: If side effects continue or become intolerable, your doctor may consider changing your prescription regimen. They can look for other antiretroviral drugs or change the dosage to reduce negative effects while maintaining successful virus suppression. Any changes, however, should be made under the supervision of a healthcare expert.

Remember that treating potential ART side effects necessitates open contact with your healthcare physician, strict adherence to drug regimens, and proactive self-care.

2.15 Holistic Wellness Approaches: Complementary Therapies and Supportive Care

Integrating holistic methods to wellness, in addition to antiretroviral medication (ART) and medical management, can improve the overall well-being of those living with HIV/AIDS. Complementary therapies and supportive care can offer additional assistance, promote physical and emotional health, and improve the overall quality of life. This section will look at various holistic approaches and their benefits for people living with HIV/AIDS.

Understanding Holistic Wellness Approaches: Holistic wellness approaches comprise a wide range of techniques that address the physical, emotional, mental, and spiritual components of health. These approaches attempt to improve people's general well-being and supplement traditional medical treatments.

Alternative Therapies: Complementary therapies are non-traditional approaches that can be utilized in addition to conventional treatments. Among the most often used complementary therapies for those living with HIV/AIDS are:

Meditation, yoga, tai chi, and deep breathing exercises: These are all mind-body techniques that can help reduce stress, increase mental clarity, and promote relaxation.

Massage therapy: It can relieve muscle tension, increase circulation, decrease anxiety, and improve general well-being.

Acupuncture: Acupuncture is the insertion of fine needles into particular spots on the body. It can help ease pain, reduce stress, and enhance overall body balance.

Herbal supplements and remedies: Certain herbs and supplements may have immune-boosting or supporting properties. However, before introducing them into your regimen, consult with a healthcare physician to ensure safety and avoid any interactions with ART.

Supportive Care: Supportive care focuses on meeting the many physical, emotional, and social needs of patients living with HIV/AIDS. It includes the following:

Palliative care: Palliative care aims to improve the quality of life by relieving pain, symptoms, and stress. It can assist patients at any stage of the disease manage physical symptoms and mental issues.

Mental health support: Such as counseling or therapy, can help people manage the emotional and psychological issues that come with living with HIV/AIDS. It offers a secure environment in which to express feelings, address concerns, and build coping mechanisms.

Nutritional counseling: Proper diet is essential for overall health and immune system support. Nutritional counseling can help you maintain a balanced diet, manage medication side effects, and address specific nutritional needs.

Social support networks, such as support groups or community organizations, can provide a sense of belonging, emotional support, and opportunities to connect with others who are experiencing similar difficulties.

Integrating Holistic Techniques: It is critical to incorporate holistic techniques into your overall healthcare plan in partnership with your healthcare professional. Discuss your interest in complementary therapies and supportive care with your doctor, and seek advice on safe and effective methods that are tailored to your specific requirements.

Precautions and safety measures: While comprehensive approaches might be advantageous, it is critical to prioritize safety. Inform your healthcare practitioner about any alternative therapies or supplements you are thinking about using to ensure they do not conflict with your ART or have any potential negative effects. Follow the instructions of skilled professionals and credible sources of information.

Self-Care and Empowerment: Holistic techniques encourage people to take an active role in their wellness journey. Self-care routines, healthy lifestyle choices, and emotional well-being can all contribute to a sense of empowerment and an enhanced quality of life.

Remember that holistic approaches to health, such as complementary therapies and supportive care, can supplement traditional medical treatments and improve the overall well-being of HIV/AIDS patients.

Chapter 3

Empowering Yourself and Creating a Supportive Network

Building a supportive network and empowering yourself are critical parts of handling pregnancy with HIV/AIDS. In this chapter, we'll look at ways to empower yourself, build a strong support system, and find resources to help you on your way to a healthy pregnancy and beyond.

3.1 Self-Empowerment: Recognizing and Embracing Your Strengths and Resilience

Recognize and embrace your inner power and resilience as you handle HIV/AIDS pregnancy. Recognize that you can overcome obstacles and make informed decisions for your own and your baby's well-being.

3.2 Empowerment via Education and Knowledge

Seek trustworthy sources of information to educate yourself on HIV/AIDS, pregnancy, and other related topics. You can make informed judgments and advocate for your requirements, as well as actively participate in your healthcare.

3.3 Self-Advocacy: Expressing Your Needs

By actively communicating your requirements to your healthcare providers, you can advocate for yourself. Proactively communicate your concerns, ask questions, and convey your preferences. Effective communication guarantees that your voice is heard and that your particular circumstances are taken into account.

3.4 Establishing a Helpful Network

Surround yourself with family, friends, and healthcare experts who understand and appreciate your experience. Look for support groups or online forums where you can connect with people going through similar experiences. Sharing one's experiences and receiving support may be both uplifting and reassuring.

3.5 Interacting with Your Partner

Communication with your spouse should be open and honest throughout the pregnancy. Share your worries, fears, and expectations Concerning HIV/AIDS and pregnancy. Develop skills for stress management, open communication, and making decisions that benefit your group's well-being.

3.6 Seeking Professional Assistance

Consider obtaining professional help from HIV/AIDS and pregnancy counselors, therapists, or social workers. They can help you manage the emotional and psychological parts of your trip by providing direction, emotional support, and practical skills.

3.7 Full disclosure: Informing Others About Your HIV Status

Make informed disclosure decisions by assessing the rewards and potential hazards. Seek advice from healthcare experts or support groups on how, when, and to whom you should reveal your HIV status. Remember that disclosure is a personal decision, and you have the right to choose what information you reveal.

3.8 Dealing with Stigma and Discrimination

Create strategies for dealing with and confronting the stigma and discrimination associated with HIV/AIDS. Learn about your rights and advocate for them. Surround yourself with people and organizations that promote diversity and combat bigotry.

3.9 Obtaining Resources and Assistance Services

Investigate the available resources and support services for HIV/AIDS and pregnancy. Prenatal care clinics, specialist healthcare providers, counseling services, financial support programs, and educational materials are examples. Using these resources can provide essential help and direction.

3.10 Wellness and Self-Care

Throughout your pregnancy, prioritize self-care and wellness. Exercise, good nutrition, relaxation techniques, and hobbies that bring you joy are all activities that improve physical, emotional, and mental well-being. Taking care of yourself benefits both you and your baby.

3.11 Empowering Others: How to Become an Advocate

Consider becoming an HIV/AIDS and pregnancy champion by sharing your experiences, increasing awareness, and fostering understanding. Your words have the potential to inspire and empower others who are facing similar circumstances.

You can navigate pregnancy with HIV/AIDS with courage, resilience, and confidence if you empower yourself, develop a supportive network, and access accessible resources. Remember that you are not alone on this journey and that by accepting your power and connecting with others, you can create a wonderful and powerful experience for yourself and your baby.

Future Planning: Preparing for Childbirth and Beyond

Childbirth and the postpartum period necessitate careful planning and consideration, especially for people living with HIV/AIDS. This chapter will go over crucial components of delivery preparation, postpartum care, and long-term planning for a healthy future.

4.1 Recognizing the Effects of HIV/AIDS on Childbirth

Learn how HIV/AIDS can affect childbirth and the steps you should take to decrease the risk of transmission to your baby. Understand the significance of sticking to your antiretroviral medication (ART) regimen and attending prenatal care sessions to achieve the best possible health results.

4.2 Working Together with Your Healthcare Team

Collaboration with your healthcare team, which includes your obstetrician, infectious disease expert, and other relevant healthcare specialists, is essential. Create a thorough strategy that covers your specific requirements and ensures you and your baby receive the finest possible care.

4.3 Selecting a Birth Plan

Investigate various birth alternatives and discuss them with your healthcare professional. Take into account your overall health, viral load, and personal preferences. Your healthcare team can help you make informed decisions about vaginal birth, cesarean section, pain management, and other aspects of childbirth.

4.4 Mother-to-Child Transmission Prevention (PMTCT)

Learn about the measures and interventions available to prevent HIV transmission from mother to child. These may include receiving antiretroviral drugs during pregnancy and labor, having an elective cesarean section in some situations, and giving your baby antiretroviral prophylaxis after birth.

4.5 Postpartum Support and Care

Get ready for the postpartum phase by comprehending the special challenges and considerations for HIV/AIDS patients. Make sure you have access to postpartum care, which includes follow-up checkups, viral load monitoring, and physical and emotional support.

4.6 Infant Feeding Alternatives

Consult your healthcare practitioner about newborn feeding alternatives to decide the best technique for you and your baby. While breastfeeding is generally not recommended for people living with HIV/AIDS, formula feeding with good sanitation and hygiene measures can be a safe option.

4.7 Family Planning and Contraception

Investigate contraception and family planning alternatives for people living with HIV/AIDS. Consult with your healthcare practitioner to choose a technique that is compatible with your reproductive objectives, provides effective contraception, and considers potential interactions with your antiretroviral medications.

4.8 Long-Term Well-Being & Health

Take preventative measures to ensure your long-term health and wellness. Maintain your ART routine, go to frequent medical check-ups, and make healthy lifestyle choices like appropriate eating, exercise, stress management, and avoiding dangerous behaviors.

4.9 Emotional and Mental Well-Being

Pay attention to your mental health and emotional well-being throughout and after pregnancy. Seek help from healthcare professionals, counselors, or support groups to deal with any difficulties or emotional issues that may occur.

4.10 Support and Parenting Systems

Create a solid support network to help you on your parenting journey. Engage with family, friends, and support groups that can offer practical help, emotional support, and advice as you negotiate the joys and challenges of raising a child while living with HIV/AIDS patients.

4.11 Your Child's Disclosure and Education

Consider when and how to tell your child about your HIV status, keeping in mind their age, maturity level, and the supportive environment you've created. Educate yourself on age-appropriate approaches to discussing HIV/AIDS with your kid to promote understanding and reduce stigma.

4.12 Future Preparation

Consider your long-term goals, such as education, profession, and financial security, while planning for the future. Investigate the resources available for people living with HIV/AIDS, such as vocational training, educational grants, and financial assistance programs that can help you achieve your goals.

You can ensure a safe and healthy experience for both you and your baby by carefully planning for childbirth and beyond. Collaboration with your healthcare team, following medical advice with the help of your network, you will contribute to a positive and empowered transition into motherhood. Remember that you have the strength and resilience to successfully navigate this chapter of your life.

Conclusion

Managing pregnancy with HIV/AIDS involves unique obstacles, but it is possible to have a healthy and satisfying journey into motherhood with the correct knowledge, support, and empowerment. Throughout this book, we have covered a variety of subjects connected to pregnancy, HIV/AIDS, and the critical considerations for people in this circumstance.

We began by learning about the impact of HIV/AIDS on pregnancy, as well as the dangers and precautions involved. We talked about the necessity of HIV testing and diagnosis during pregnancy, treatment options, and the implications of drug management and treatment adherence. We also discussed how to manage health and well-being during pregnancy, such as self-care, mental well-being, nutrition, exercise, and avoiding opportunistic infections.

Furthermore, we investigated the value of developing a supporting network, eliminating stigma, and overcoming disclosure barriers as well as incorporating partners in the pregnancy process. Prenatal care, regular monitoring, and supporting healthy mental health and coping methods were all highlighted. We also talked about pregnancy and family planning options, as well as sexual and reproductive health education and counseling.

Furthermore, we emphasized the treatment of probable antiretroviral therapy (ART) adverse effects, holistic approaches to wellness, and empowering oneself while developing a support system. We talked about prenatal care, postpartum care, and long-term planning for a healthy future.

Individuals can face the obstacles of HIV/AIDS pregnancy with courage, resilience, and confidence by taking proactive efforts such as educating themselves, advocating for needs, and using accessible resources and support services. It is critical to remember that self-advocacy, open communication with healthcare practitioners, and the assistance of a strong network are critical components of this trip.

As we come to the end of this book, we want to underline how unique each person's experience with HIV/AIDS and pregnancy is. When making decisions concerning medical treatment, lifestyle choices, and disclosure, it is critical to speak with healthcare professionals who specialize in this sector and to consider specific circumstances.

Finally, we want to express our love, encouragement, and admiration to anyone embarking on the road of pregnancy with HIV/AIDS. You are strong, resilient, and capable of overcoming obstacles. You can create a positive and fulfilling experience for yourself and your baby by keeping informed, seeking help, and embracing self-care and empowerment.

Keep in mind that you are not alone on this path. With the proper information, resources, and tools. With our help, you may navigate an HIV/AIDS pregnancy and embrace the joy and beauty of becoming a parent while prioritizing your health and the well-being of your child. May this book be a beneficial guide and companion on your journey to a healthy and satisfying HIV/AIDS pregnancy!